Arthritis Pain Relief Naturally

By Edgar Ortega M.

What is Arthritis?

I 'm sure everyone either knows someone who has arthritis or has at least heard of it.

Basically, the definition of arthritis is the inflammation of one or more of your joints, and it is used to describe over 100 different conditions and diseases that affect joints, tissues around joints, as well as other connective tissues.

"But I'm not that old so I can't have arthritis!" Although it's common that adults 65 and older are affected by arthritis, it can also affect people of ALL ages, ethnic groups, and races.

A shocking statistic shows that approximately 1 out of 5 adults (about 50 million people) in the United States have been diagnosed by their doctors with some type of arthritis.

There are two common forms of arthritis, osteoarthritis arthritis and rheumatoid arthritis.

Types of Arthritis

Osteoarthritis arthritis

This is the most common form of arthritis in the United States.

Often referred to as "wear and tear arthritis," osteoarthritis (OA) affects approximately 27 million Americans. It is also sometimes called degenerative joint disease or degenerative arthritis most commonly affective people older than 65.

What does osteoarthritis do? It breaks downs the cartilage that covers the ends of the bones. This important cartilage is what forms a joint and allows movement.

Over time as the cartilage wears away, the bones become exposed and without the cartilage to protect the ends, the bones rub against each other.

This deterioration of cartilage affects the shape of the joint so that it no longer functions as it should.

There are other problems that may take place in the joint itself.

The breakdown of cartilage can affect the joint components.

This is where fragments of cartilage or bone may float in joint fluid, causing not only irritation but pain as well.

Osteophytes, or spurs, can develop at the ends of the bones.

This damages the tissues that surround the bones also causing pain.

Hyaluronan, a substance found in the fluid that is inside the joint, might affect the ability of the joint to absorb shock.

To make matters worse, inflammation may also occur in the lining of the joint, due to the cartilage breakdown.

Rheumatoid Arthritis

Rheumatoid arthritis (RA) is similar to osteoarthritis, where they both affect the joints.

But the difference is that RA is an autoimmune disease where the body's immune system, which normally Supposed to protect our bodies from infection by attacking viruses and bacteria, attacks normal joint tissues, causing inflammation of the joint lining.

As of writing this, no one fully understands why it happens, but for some reason rheumatoid arthritis causes the immune system to go haywire and attacks healthy cells such as the synovium.

Snovium is a very important thin membrane that lines the joints. This attack causes fluid buildup in the joints which can cause pain, stiffness, inflammation, warmth, and redness.

Over time the cartilage wears away, the joint loses its shape, and bones erode, affecting not only function but mobility as well.

Because of this, the inflammation then affects organs such as the skin, eyes, blood, heart, and lungs.

RA is an ongoing disease, with flares (active periods of pain and inflammation) that disappears and reappears randomly.

What does rheumatoid arthritis affect?

It most commonly affects the joints of the hands, wrists, elbows, knees, feet, and ankles. If one joint gets affected then the same joint on the other side or opposite side of the body is affected as well.

There is no single laboratory test that can confirm a diagnosis of RA.

If your doctor suspects you might have rheumatoid arthritis, the first thing that must be done to take your medical history to gather specific information about your symptoms.

Some questions that might be asked include: Do you have pain in several joints? Do you experience stiffness in the morning? Are you often fatigued?

The doctor will then give you a physical exam looking for swelling, warmth, tenderness, limited motion in your joints, or nodules under the skin.

Currently, this disease has no cure and the symptoms often come and go.

If your doctor has diagnosed you with RA, you are not alone. This disease affects approximately 1.5 million people in the United States.

Also three times more women are affected then men.

Although it can begin at any age, even as a child, the usual age for adults are between the ages of 40 and 60 years old.

Signs and Symptoms

Osteoarthritis arthritis

Symptoms of osteoarthritis usually develop slowly.

There may be soreness or stiffness at first that seems more like an annoyance than a medical issue.

For some, the first signs of OA are joints that ache after exercise or physical work.

As the disease progresses, the most common symptoms are:

- Pain in a joint

- Swelling or tenderness in one or more joints

- Stiffness after resting that goes away after movement

- Flare-ups of pain and inflammation after use of the affected joint

- Crunching feeling or sound of bone rubbing on bone (called crepitus) when the joint is used.

- Sore or stiff joints - particularly the hips, knees, and lower back—after inactivity or overuse

- Pain that is worse after activity or toward the end of the day.

Osteoarthritis may also affect the small finger joints, the neck, the base of the thumb, ankle, and big toe.

The pain may come and go, without affecting the ability to perform daily tasks.

Some people who Suffer from OA will never progress past this early stage.

Others will have their OA get worse as time progresses. Some may have the pain and stiffness be so severe that it may make it difficult to walk, climb stairs, sleep, or perform other daily tasks.

OA most often occurs in the following areas:

Knees

Knees are joints that are considered weight-bearing joints.

Because of this, they are very commonly affected by OA.

If you have OA in your knees, you may feel that these joints are stiff, sometimes swollen, and painful, making it difficult to walk, climb, and get in and out of things such as chairs and bathtubs.

Patients may develop a limp which can get worse as more cartilage deteriorates.

Severe osteoarthritis of the knees is one of the most common reasons for total knee replacement Surgery in the United States.

Hip?

If you have OA in the hip, you may experience pain, stiffness, and severe disability, since hips both support the weight of the body and allow movement of your lower body.

When you have OA in your hips, you may feel the pain in your groin, inner thigh, or even your knees.

Similarly to having OA in your knees, OA in the hip can also lead to difficulty moving, bending, and walking.

Spine

OA can also affect your spine. You may experience stiffness and pain in the lower back or even in the neck.

Sometimes arthritis-related changes in the spine may put pressure on the nerves, which may cause weakness or numbness in either your arms or legs.

Fingers and Hands

When OA attacks the hands and fingers, the base of the thumb joint is usually affected and people suffer with stiffness, numbness, and aching. Other symptoms of hand and finger OA include:

- Heberden's nodes: small bony knobs that appear on the end joints of fingers

- Bouchards's nodes: small bony knobs that appear on the middle joints of fingers

Rheumatoid arthritis

Rheumatoid arthritis (RA) is a chronic or long term autoimmune disease where the body's immune system attacks normal joint tissues, causing inflammation of the joint lining.

Some people experience long periods of remission, where they have few or no symptoms during this time, while other people
might have almost constant RA symptoms for months at a time.

Symptoms of Rheumatoid Arthritis

As rheumatoid arthritis attacks the joints, they become inflamed this is usually the body's natural response to infections. If you experience some of these symptoms, you may want to talk to your doctor:

- Stiffness. This is where the joint becomes harder to use and the range of motion is limited. A hallmark symptom of rheumatoid arthritis is "morning stiffness." Pain and stiffness lasts for more than 1 hour (sometimes several hours) in the morning before their joints feel loose.

- Swelling. As fluid enters the joint, it becomes puffy causing and accompanying the stiffness.

- Pain. Inflammation occurs inside a joint making rt tender and sensitive. As the inflammation continues it will cause damage contributing to pain.

- Redness. The joints that are being affected may become warmer and red-
  der than the Surrounding skin.

- Joints. The joints that are almost always affected are hands, knees, wrists,
  neck, shoulders, feet, elbows, hips, and the jaw.

The inflammation caused by RA leads to a wide variety of symptoms that affect the entire body such as fatigue, fever, malaise (general sense of not feeling well), appetite loss, and muscle aches.

Some of the symptoms of moderate to severe rheumatoid arthritis include:

• Rheumatoid nodules. Rheumatoid nodules are small lumps that develop under the skin which vary in size and often appear on the elbows. About 25% of the people with RA Suffer from this symptom which can sometimes be painful.

• Lungs. Due to the damage of the lungs or inflammation of the lining surrounding the lungs, shortness of breath may develop.

This can be treated with certain drugs which can reduce the inflammation.

Cricoarytenoid Joint Also known as the voice box or larynx. RA can affect this joint causing hoarseness.

Eyes.

Some people (approximately 5%) with RA may experience symptoms in the eyes include red, painful and sometimes dry eyes.
You may also feel shortness of breath or chest pain do to inflammation in the lining around the heart.

Also, people with rheumatoid arthritis may develop clogged arteries in their heart which can lead to chest pain and even a heart attack.

Causes

Osteoarthritis arthritis

Years ago doctors used to tell their patients that OA is brought on by joints that have simply worn out due to old age.

But research has led to a better understanding of osteoarthritis which determined that there are distinct subtypes, called phenotypes. Each phenotype has its own risk factors.

Genetics

As of writing this, there have been three genes that are linked to a higher risk of developing OA.

Genetic Susceptibility to osteoarthritis is complex, where each gene that plays a role contributes only a modest amount to the susceptibility.

Currently, there are no major impact genes for OA.

Research is still being done and there are no interventions that exist for genetic abnormalities in regards to OA.

In the future, doctors hope to offer people some
kind of risk prediction based on their genetic profile.

Post Traumatic

Researchers have determined that 50% of people will develop a form of osteoarthritis 10 to 20 years after a traumatic injury to the knee, such as an ACL
or meniscus tear.

This complicated process involves a chain reaction of changes in the joint that take place as the body's natural repair process desperately attempts to keep up with the biological and chemical changes that happen in response to the injury.

Whether OA develops or not is based on numerous factors such as genetic variability, gender (women have a greater risk), age (older at the time of injury have a higher risk), body mass index
(BMI), and the type of injury.

Researchers are trying to find a way to interferewith those chemical changes that occur after a trauma.

- Cartilage acts as a shock absorber, allowingthe joint to move smoothly.

- As cartilage breaks down, the ends of the bones thicken and the joint may lose its normal shape.

- With further cartilage breakdown, the ends of the bones may begin to rub together, causing pain.

- In addition, damaged joint tissue can cause the release of certain substances called prostaglandins, which can also contribute to the pain and swelling characteristic of the disease.

Obesity

Why would obesity affect your risk of getting OA? One reason is biomechanical, where being overweight or obese is more taxing on your joints.

Obesity also affects non-weight bearing joints such as in the hand.

This occurs when fat tissue releases chemicals that increase inflammation thus affecting
the joints.

One study found that higher levels of leptin were related to the narrowing of joint space in the hip.

This is an early sign of arthritis.

Studies are still being done on other chemicals released by fat tissue, such as estrogen and adiponectin.

Age

Getting older is the greatest risk factor for Osteoarthritis. Although aging does not directly cause OA, but 50 percent of people older than 65 do have it.

According to Dr. Richard Loeser, program director of both the Translational Science Institute and the Sticht Center on Aging at Wake Forest University School of Medicine in Winston-Salem, N.C., genes, prior injury, obesity, and aging contributes to the development of OA because of the changes that occur to the joint(s) overtime.

Why don't all older adults get OA? Researchers still don't know.

They believe that OA is related to abnormal mechanical stress caused by

injury or misaligned joints, not the normal or everyday loading on joints. According to a
Dutch study that took 80 adults, aged 89 to 91, which found that 63 percent had no hip OA, 51 percent had no knee OA, and 29 percent had no hand OA.

They found that men were least likely to develop OA.

Unfortunately there is currently no way to stop or slow down the aging process.

Rheumatoid arthritis

The answer is still not clear, but most doctors agree that a combination of genetic and environmental factors may be responsible.

But research has shewn that several factors may contribute to the development of RA:

Sex

Women are more likely than others to have this disease.

Women with rheumatoid arthritis outnumber men three to one.

According to the American College of Rheumatology, 3 percent of women may get RA in their lifetime.

Age

RA affects older teenagers and adults of all ages.

Younger teens and children may also be diagnosed with a related form called juvenile idiopathic
arthritis.

Usually, it begins in women that are between the ages of 30 and 60, where as in men it often occurs later on in life.

Family

The majority of people who Suffer from RA have no family history of the disease.

But researchers say that having a family member with Rheumatoid arthritis increases the odds of having it.

Genetic

Certain genes play a role in the immune system.

For some people, genetic factors may be involved in determining whether or not they will have rheumatoid arthritis.

Some research shows that people with a genetic marker called
the HLA shared epitope have 5 times the risk of having rheumatoid arthritis compared to people without the marker.

Signal transducer and activator of transcription 4 (STAT4) and protein tyrosine phosphatase, non-receptor type 22 (PTPN22) are other genes that increase the risk of developing RA.

These genes are involved in other autoimmune diseases in some people.

Obesity

In a recent study by the researchers at the Mayo Clinic found that people who are obese are 25 percent more likely to have RA than people with normal weight.

Smoking

In 2010 a Swedish study found that smoking may be responsible for as many as 1 in 5 cases of rheumatoid arthritis overall and a larger percent of cases in people that have positive blood tests for anti-citrullinated protein antibodies, this is an antibody that is associated with more severe RA.

The suggest that a person's risk of RA varies based upon how much and how long they smoke, but for heavy smokers there is an increased risk even 20 years after quitting.

Osteoarthritis treatments

Surgical. Most people who Suffer from osteoarthritis will never need Surgery, but if they Suffer from severe joint damage, extreme pain, or very limited motion as a result of this condition, than osteoarthritis surgery might be necessary.

Surgery helps the patient by replacing the damaged joint with a synthetic one that can allow one to continue activities that they enjoy.

Also surgically replacing the painful joint or even removing loose growths that are causing pain can relieve pain.

Surgery can also be used if the joint becomes maligned so that it no longer functions as it should and/or it looks unusual.

Hip replacement Surgery, joint fusion Surgery, joint replacement Surgery, and knee replacement Surgery should be discussed with your doctor to see if you

are an
acceptable candidate for these
treatments.

Medications for Osteoarthritis

The medications used to treat arthritis
vary depending on the type of arthritis.

Commonly used arthritis medications
include:

Analgesics

These types of medications help reduce
pain, but have no effect on inflammation.

Examples include acetaminophen (Tylenol,
others), tramadol (Ultram, Ryzolt, others)
and narcotics containing oxycodone
(Percocet, Oxycontin, others) or
hydrocodone (Vicodin, Lortab, others).

The American College of Rheumatology
recommends that acetaminophen be used
for the treatment of mild or moderate pain
caused by osteoarthritis. Do not take more
than 3000mg/day unless otherwise
directed by your doctor.

For chronic pain, you be prescribed
hydrocodone or other opioids which are

also used to ease severe, acute pain after joint Surgery or a bone fracture due to osteoporosis.

Nonsteroidal anti-inflammatory drugs (NSAIDs)

NSAIDs reduce both pain and inflammation.

Over-the-counter NSAIDs include ibuprofen (Advil, Motrin IB, others) and naproxen (Aleve). Some types of NSAIDs are available only by prescription. Some NSAIDs are also available as creams or gels, which can be rubbed on joints.

Some of these drugs have been linked to an increase in gastrointestinal bleeding, stomach ulcers, hearth attack and stroke.

Connterirritants

Some varieties of creams and ointments contain menthol or capsaicin, the ingredient that makes hot peppers spicy.

Rubbing these preparations on the skin over your aching joint may interfere with the transmission of pain signals from the joint itself.

Some examples of these include brand names such as ArthriCare, Eucalyptamint, Icy Hot and Therapeutic Mineral Ice, among others.

A type of NSAID is called Voltaren Gel. Available only by prescription, this gel is recommended by the American College of Rheumatology that people over the age of 75 use this topical NSAID instead of those taken by the mouth.

Disease-modifying antirheumatic drugs (DMARDs). Often used to treat rheumatoid arthritis, DMARDs slow or stop your immune System from attacking your joints.

Examples include methotrexate (Trexall) and hydroxychloroquine (Plaquenil). Biologic?

Typically used in conjunction with DMARDs, biologic response modifiers are genetically engineered drugs that target various protein molecules that are involved in the immune response.

Examples include etanercept (Enbrel) and infliximab (Remicade).

Corticosteroids

This class of drug, which includes prednisone and cortisone, reduces inflammation and suppresses the immune system. They are powerful anti-inflammatory medicines that are often prescribed for people with arthritis that need a quick relief from severe inflammation.

The American College of Rheumatology recommends that corticosteroid injections be used as an alternate therapy for people who have moderate to severe knee pain with signs of inflammation that are not feeling better after taking acetaminophen.

Corticosteroids can be taken orally or be injected directly into the painful joint.

These injections can be taken in the same joint 3 to 4 times per year.

Hyaluronic acid therapy

Hyaluronic acid is found naturally in joint fluid, where it is used as a shock absorber and lubricant. However, in people with osteoarthritis the acid appears to break down.

By injecting hyaluronic acid (Synvisc, Hyalgan) into the joint, it may help lessen pain and inflammation.

According to ACR guidelines, hyaluronic acid therapy may help patients with knee OA that are not feeling better using NSAIDs, or for those who have had adverse side effects from these drugs.

Top Ten Non-Drug Treatments for Osteoarthritis

1. Regular telephone contact. The best evidence for the benefit of phone contact came from a study of 439 OA patients. Here the patients received monthly phone calls from lay personnel promoting self-care which showed improvements in joint pain and physical function for up to a year.

2. Physical therapy. Studies consistently support the effectiveness of an evaluation

by a physical therapist and instruction in suitable exercises to reduce pain and improve function. Physical therapists can provide devices to make daily tasks easier.

1. Aerobic, muscle-strengthening and water-based exercises. A well rounded exercise program can not only promote muscle strength, but improve
range of motion, increase mobility and ease pain as well.

2. Weight loss. Maintaining your recommended weight or losing weight if
you are overweight can lessen your pain by reducing stress on the affected joints. As mentioned earlier, weight loss helps ease pressure on weight-bearing joints such as the hips and knees.

3. Walking aids. Canes and crutches can reduce pain in hip and knee or OA. Wheeled walkers may be used if both hips and/or knees are affected.

4. Footwear and insoles. Special footwear and insoles can be used if

osteoarthritis affects the knee. This can help reduce pain and improve walking.

5. Knee braces. For osteoarthritis with associated knee instability, a knee brace can reduce pain, improve Stability and reduce risks of falling.

6. Heat and cold. Many patients find that the heat of a warm bath, heat pack or paraffin bath eases their OA pain. Others find relief in cold packs, while others prefer alternating the two.

Electrical nererve simulation

(TENS). TENS is a technique in which a weak electric current is administered through elec-
trodes placed on the skin. TENS is believed to stop messages from pain receptors from reaching the brain. Studies show that it is effective in helping with short-term pain control in some patients with knee or hip arthritis.

1. Acupuncture. This is a form of traditional Chinese medicine where

thin, sharp needles are inserted at specific points on the body.

2. Acupuncture
   has been used as a treatment for osteoarthritis pain. A recent trial of 352
   patients with knee osteoarthritis showed small but statistically significant improvement in pain intensity 2 and 4 weeks after a course of acupuncture.

Medications for Rheumatoid Arthritis

There are many different drugs used in the treatment of rheumatoid arthritis.

Some are used primarily to ease the symptoms of RA where as others are used to slow or stop the course of the disease and to inhibit structural damage.

Most of these drugs fall into one of the following categories:

The following treatments are the same as those for Osteoarthritis
NSAIDs: Similar to osteoarthritis treatments, NSAIDs can be used. NSAIDs include such drugs as ibuprofen (Advil, Motrin), ketoprofen (Actron, Orudis KT) arc raproxer sociur-i (Aleve), ariorg o:rers. If you rave hac or are a: risk of stomach ulcers, your doctor may prescribe celecoxib (Celebrex), a type of NSAID called a COX-2 inhibitor, which is designed to be safer for the stomach.

Corticosteroids - Corticosteroid medications, including prednisone, prednisolone and methyprednisolone, are potent and quick-acting anti- inflam-inflammatory medications. They may be used in RA to get potentially damaging inflammation under control, while waiting for NSAIDs and DMARDs (below) take effect.

DMARDs: Acronyms for disease-modifying antirheumatic drugs, DMARDs
are drugs that work slowly to actually modify the course of the disease.

The most commonly used DMARD for rheumatoid arthritis is methotrexate.

Others
that fall into this category and they include hydroxycholorquine (Plaquenil), sulfasalazine (Azulfidine, Azulfidine EN-Tabs), leflunomide (Arava) and azathioprine (Imuran).

A person diagnosed with rheumatoid arthritis today is likely to be prescribed a DMARD fairly early in the course of their disease, as doctors have found that starting these drugs early on can help prevent the irreparable joint damage that might occur if the use of this drug was delayed.

Biologic agents: Biologic response modifiers, or biologies are a subset of DMARDs.

There are currently nine such agents approved for rheumatoid arthritis: abatacept (Orencia), adalimumab (Humira), anakinra (Kineret), cer-tolizumab pegol (Cimzia) etanercept (Enbrel), infliximab (Remicade), goli-mumab (Simponi) and rituximab (Rituxan).

Each of the biologies blocks a specific step in the inflammation process.

Cimzia, Enbrel, Humira, Remicade and Simponi block a cytokine called tumor necrosis factor-alpha (TNF), and therefore often are called TNF inhibitors.

Kineret blocks a cytokine called interleukin-1 (IL-1), Orencia blocks the activation of T cells, Rituxan blocks B cells, and Actemra blocks a cytokine called interleukin-6 (IL-6).

Since these agents target specific steps in the process, they do not destroy the entire immune response as some other RA treatments do. In fact many people find that a biologic agent can slow, modify or stop the disease – even when other treatments haven't helped much.

JAK inhibitors: This is a new drug, tofacitinib (Xeljanz) which is being compared to biologies. However, it is part of a new subcategory of DMARDs known as JAK inhibitors that block Janus kinase, or JAK, pathways, which are in-volved in the body's immune response.

Nutrients that can help with OA

SAM-e (S-adenosylmethionine). This synthetic form of a chemical found in all human cells is a natural analgesic and anti-inflammatory that may stimulate cartilage growth by signaling production of cartilage proteins.

A 2004 University of California, Irvine study found SAM-e equal to the prescription drug celecoxib (Celebrex) and a 2009 study found it comparable to the NSAID nabumetone. It also has fewer side effects!

Folic acid, or folate, is a B vitamin that helps your body make red blood cells.

If you are prescribed the drug methotrexate, folic acid may help you to avoid some of the drug's side effects.

Supplementing your diet with bone-boosting calcium and vitamin D is important, especially if you take corticosteroids (like prednisone) that can cause bone loss.

Check with your doctor to see how much calcium and vitamin D you need to get daily through foods. Supplements, and sunlight.

Omega-3 fatty acids are found in fish such as salmon, tuna, and trout; walnuts; tofu and other soybean products; flaxseed and flaxseed oil; and
canola oil. They are known to help reduce inflammation. Fish oil supplements also contain omega-3 fatty acids. According to the American

College of Rheumatology, some people with RA report less pain and joint tenderness when taking it.

You may not notice immediate results, in fact it may take weeks or months to feel a difference.

A 2010 meta-analysis found that fish oil significantly decreased joint tenderness and stiffness
in RA patients and reduced or eliminated NSAID use.

Boswellia serrata (Indian frankincense) is a gum resin of the boswellia tree.

It has strong anti-inflammatory and analgesic properties that may
help prevent cartilage loss and inhibit the autoimmune process.

Try to fire a procuc::r-a: cor:airs a: <v\: 60 percer: boswellic acics arc :ake 300 to 400 mg three times daily.

Capsaicin (Capsicum frutescens) is the active, heat producing component in chili peppers. It temporarily reduces substance P, a pain transmitter.

A study published in Phytotherapy Research in 2010 found that
joint pain decreased almost 50 percent after three weeks of use of 0.05 percent capsaicin cream.

Turmeric/curcumin (Curcuma longa) is the root of a plant in the ginger family that when used can block inflammatory cytokines and enzymes, including cyclooxygenase-2 (COX-2), the target of celecoxib. A 2010 clin-
ical trial found that a turmeric Supplement called Meriva (standardized to 75 percent curcumin combined with phosphatidylcholine) provided longterm improvement in pain and function in 100

patients with knee OA. Also a small 2012 pilot study, a curcumin product called BCM-95 reduced

joint pain and swelling in patients with active RA better than diclofenac sodium did. 500 mg two to four times a day for OA and 500 mg twice daily for RA.

Avocado-soybean unsaponifiables (ASU) is a supplement composed of l/3rC* avocado oil and 2/3rC* soybean oil. IT works by blocking proinflammatory chemicals which prevents deterioration of synovial cells that line joints and help regenerate normal connective tissues.

A 2008 meta-analysis found that ASU improved symptoms of hip and knee OA and reduced or eliminated NSAID use.

Nutrients that can help with RA

Cat's claw (Uncaria tomentosa) is the bark and root of South American vine.

This is an anti-inflammatory that inhibits tumor necrosis factor
(TNF) and contains compounds that may benefit the immune system.

A trial in 2002 showed that it it reduced joint pain and swelling by more than 50 percent compared with placebo.

Whether you get it by capsule,
tablet, tea, or extract, try taking 60 mg daily in divided doses.
Fish oil from cold-water fish such as salmon and herring. This has a rich source of the omega-3 fatty acids EPA and DHA.

EPA and DHA have been studied for RA and other inflammatory conditions. A 2010 metaanalysis found that fish oil significantly decreased joint tenderness and stiffness in RA patients and reduced or eliminated NSAID use.

Use 3.8 grams EPA and 2 grams DHA daily for RA. Try to find brands that have 85 percent to 90 percent concentrations of omega-3s.
GLA (gamma linolenic acid) is an omega-6 fatty acid that is found in some plant-seed oils, including borage, black currant, and evening primrose.

The body converts GLA into anti-inflammatory chemicals. In a 2005 trial of 56 patients with active RA, they found significant improvement in joint pain, stiffness and grip strength after six months and progressive
improvement in control of disease activity at one year. Whether you take a capsule, oil. or softgel, take 300 mg to 3 grams daily in divided doses or 450 mg GLA and 240 mg EPA daily.

- Ginger (Zingiber officinale) has been shown to have a anti-inflammatory properties similar to ibuprofen and COX-2 inhibitors. In 2012 an in vitro study found that a specialized ginger extract called Eurovita Extract 77 reduced inflammatory reactions in RA synovial cells as effectively as steroids did. Take 255 mg of Eurovita Extract 77 twice daily.

– Talk to your doctor before taking any supplements. Your doctor can check on
the dose you need, since the dose used in medical studies was much higher
than what you'd get from a normal supplement without a prescription.

6 Foods to Avoid

- Researchers at the Mount Sinai
  School of Medicine found that
  cutting
  back on the consumption of fried
  and processed foods, can reduce
  inflammation and actually help
  restore the body's natural defenses.

- Eat less fried and processed foods
  and include more vegetables and
  fruits in your diet.

- Keep your Sugars and Refined Carbs
  Low

- High amounts of sugar in the diet
  can result in inflammation

- Cut out candies, processed foods,
  white flour baked goods, and sodas
  to
  reduce arthritis

1. Dairy Products

- According to the Physicians Committee for Responsible Medicine, for
  some people this protein may irritate the tissue around the joints.

- Get protein from sources like vegetables such as spinach, nut butters, tofu, beans, lentils, and quinoa.

- Tobacco and Alcohol. Tobacco and alcohol use can affect your joints.

- Cut back on drinking and ramp up healthy eating habits, regular exercise,
  and good quality sleep

- Salt and Preservatives

- Many foods contain excessive salt and other preservatives to promote longer shelf lives, but excess consumption of salt may result in inflammation of the joints.

- Avoid prepared meals.

- Most microwavable meals are very high in sodium

- Corn Oil

- Baked goods and snacks contain corn or other oils high in omega-6 fatty
  acids which may trigger inflammation.

Instead of foods containing omega-6 fatty acids use healthy, anti-infiaminflammatory omega-3 alternatives such as olive oil, nuts, flax seeds, and pumpkin seeds.

Alternative Treatments

Exercise

Exercises and physical therapy can help improve the range of motion as well as strengthen the muscles Surrounding the joints.
Acupuncture

As mentioned previously, acupuncture can be used for treatment of arthri-tis. Although it is not a "cure-all" treatment, it can be effective in treating chronic pain such as arthritis, low back, neck, or muscle pain, and pain after surgery. During the acupuncture treatment, the acupuncturist will swab each acu-point area with alcohol to sanitize the area before inserting a hair-thin, metal needle into the site. They are placed under the skin in carefully calculated points. The number of needles varies based upon the treatment. They stay in place for a few minutes to an hour. During this time the needles are twirled, energized electrically, or warmed.

Aromatherapy

Aromatherapy is the therapeutic use of scented essential oils. You can inhale the oils, use them in the bath or massage them into your skin. When you use them for massage they're diluted in carrier oil.

There are many different oils you can use. An aromatherapist might select lavender or marjoram to relieve muscle spasm, or ginger if you have a circulatory problem. The oils are very concentrated and you should never apply

them to your skin undiluted. Many people with pain report that an aromatherapy massage gives relief for several weeks.

Homeopathy

Homeopathy is a form of treatment founded by Samuel Hahnemann in the 18th century.

The Society of Homeopaths states that homeopathy is based on the theory of'treating like with like' and an observation that symptoms of an illness are identical to those experienced by a healthy person treated for that illness.

Homeopathic remedies are produced by diluting (watering down) an active substance that causes similar symptoms in the belief that this will reduce
the likelihood of harm.

This is practiced by professional homeopaths who are
qualified to prescribe remedies according to their diagnosis.

Osteopathy

Osteopathy, also known as osteopathic medicine, was founded by Dr Andrew Taylor Still, an American physician in the 19th century.

Its philosophy gives a holistic approach to health and stresses the importance of the muscu-
loskeletal system in a person's health and well-being. The aim of treatment is to support the body's self-healing capacity.

An osteopath centers on your whole body, including the soft tissues (such as muscles, ligaments and tendons), the spine and nervous system, and may use a variety of different hands on methods.

Since this technique uses a gentle approach, it can be suitable for many different people from newborn to the elderly, and also for those with complex medical problems.

www.ingramcontent.com/pod-product-compliance
Lightning Source LLC
Chambersburg PA
CBHW070625290526
45790CB00002B/1000